Prologue

Death, before going to the other life, invites me to tea and I wonder:

-"Why waste your time on a necessary task, a struggle as magnificent as it is irrelevant?" The fact of postponing life does not mean defeating death. Do you think you are useful? Do you think you will frustrate my works, that you will compete with me? I will always win. Sooner or later, I will leave you as inept in front of everyone, as the culprit of what happened. You are given a single opportunity and instead of using it, you come to commit suicide, to torture your soul. Study all your life to dedicate yours to see the worst of it. It has no logic! Why Medicine?

I took a sip of that tea that didn't taste like anything and answered:

-Don't expect me to think logically… I've fallen in love.

Diagnosis: body city

Tell me about my body before going to sleep. How is the life of the cells? If our organism were from a world, what would it be like? low I read in books, but I can't understand it nor did I have to make this reality. Can you imagine something similar? What do you think that city would be called, dad?

The perfect society some called it. A place where everyone knew his position and the reason for his existence. A dictatorship of the subconscious implanted by the laws of DNA. A barrier against pathological empires called skin and formed by fallen soldiers. A highly specialized security service with difficult core training. A neural aristocracy responsible for thought. Great trams that would recover enormous distances from scalp to toe. Trading blood cells that sold oxygen for CO2. A great liver industry, innumerable digestive ports, thermoelectric plants capable of keeping a nation lit without resting for a single moment. Too much responsibility for a handful of people. A world full of balance and a society as fair as it is utopian, but, as we all know, any perfect society is turned into hell by the human being.

Diagnosis: skin

—Why study Dermatology?

—I suppose it's because I love the architecture of certain walls.

«What will be beyond the wall?», a melanocyte wondered from his guard post. "It is said that we will die if we go out." So said my father, who is now part of the great protective structure. It is an honor for every melanocyte to protect it, a pride for our generations. Every time we die, we are part of the skin, protecting our nation from external threats, from invaders, from extreme temperatures. What will be in other parts of the body? Will they stand guard until death just like us? I better not think about it; the last one to do so developed into a melanoma and was killed. In fact, I heard that in another body one triumphed and went everywhere, although his republic fell. I better continue guard, although doubts torment me.

Diagnosis: body defense system

"How is the body protected?"

—Every nation, in order to exist, will need an army. Our He is despotic, narcissistic, willing to do anything...

The Core Central Command, among its functions, had to train a despotic, cold army, faithful to its governmental cause. Since they were children they practiced brainwashing. What greater pride than fighting for your skin? They had several divisions, each specialized in its field. The lymphocytes were in charge of torturing the rapists, viruses that penetrated the cells without permission and destroyed them to reproduce. The leukocytes were as cold as the serial killers they faced, while the psychopathic macrophages for hire were created by the government to clean up the mess, both external and internal. The dendritic detectives were in charge of investigating everyone who arrived and informing the Government in case they represented a threat. The eosinophils controlled the parasites of society, swindlers, beings who lived off gambling and vice. Mast cells created a large-scale, conspicuous displacement called inflammation, and closed off an area in order to kill the enemy. It was a system created with the aim of eliminating any threat, regardless of the losses.

Diagnosis: neurons

—If neurons were people, what would they be like?

—True leaders, devoted to the point of never resting, scarce as in our world today...

The great aristocrats, undisputed leaders who electrified the masses with their speeches, worked tirelessly day and night to maintain homeostasis. The myelin layers represented their royalty, those unique and irreplaceable beings were worth millions of cells. As skilled as they were weak, they could not miss their glucose delicacy, since the good life prevented them from going hungry. Some were artists, others mathematicians, all kinds of people, executioners, poets, meteorologists, visionaries, critics, craftsmen, musicians, great strategists, sensitive as themselves. Protected like no one else, their security was unmatched, it was a Council of State, an elitist leadership.

Diagnosis: lung

-"If the lung stopped breathing, what would happen, Dad?"

—It would be the economic fall of our republic. It's the bank most unusual on Earth.

The Federal Reserve in an organ, gaseous gold, the streets of Wall Street through the alveoli. With a stock market built on saturation, white-coated statesmen couldn't predict an economic meltdown or frenzied development, as the stock market system changed by the second. The cells trembled when you submerged in the water and party when meditating in the forest. The Government had a pact that was as obligatory as it was natural: it bought the gold with the CO_2 from the plants, developed its economy and collected taxes from the cells for using such a precious resource. CO_2 was the only currency the Botanical Government accepted. Many bankers walked by without knowing that cigarettes closed branches, that microorganisms stole millions, that it was necessary to sow more partners.

Diagnosis: heart

—Quick, dad, tell me, what is the heart?

—The powerhouse of our body.

The representation of the will, a chemical game that created electricity from nothing against all probability, a fist that hits you showing that it can be done, four cavities that teach you that all great work is by stage, valves that indicate that, if you want pump well, you need to take a break. Someone like him gets a lot of attention, someone like him gets a lot of abuse. «I will beat to death..., they need me». It is the politics of aid, the strongest reason that exists. It feeds after helping the body, the coronaries have their function very clear. A leader like no one else, he made arteries and veins work, different extremes that make excellence working together. I remember the phrase of the sinus node before inaugurating it: «Create electricity at all costs, as if you have to unite anions with cations. Find a way for this heart to beat. A child's life depends on us."

Diagnosis: kidneys

—If the kidney were a country, what would it be?

—If the world were flat, this would be the limit. if i were a city, it would be Venice.

The science of the body, a complex network of channels, the aquatic world. Many substances go on a tour by taking pictures of the glomeruli and ducts. Visas are granted to a few to enter and exit. You can travel and return, you can travel and lose yourself in nothingness, it is the corner where the world ends. The waters turn murky if you stop drinking, ensuring illegal entry for infectious divers. It is both channel and prey, a moon that regulates the bodily tide. It presents its embassy in the heart, great pacts with red blood cells and an unstable contract with hypertension. It's too much power for a province, decide what to remove, the acid or the basic, the electrolytes or the water. It is the executioner of urea, the purifier of life.

Diagnosis: tongue

«Language has been the richest of the human being, and within the richest, language has been the worst of this species» (phrase that a tutor always said).

The strongest musculature in a very problematic area, the flavor of a lifetime and the pang that precedes death, that is the tongue. It is as sweet as a flattery, as bitter as the truth, as acid as criticism, as salty as tears, the doctorate of the kiss and the alternative that sex leaves. It has great irrigation so as not to skimp on words, and it doesn't matter if they are lies or truth, or if they will save a life or not, it is a cursed organ. It resists being still, to remain in the mouth, and sleeps in the sky displaying its power. It is a spear made up of tissues full of taste buds, killing silence every time it feels like it.

Diagnosis: microbiota

There are qualities as good as immoral; there are assassins necessary to maintain a life.

It was a necessary evil, the price of freedom according to some, a mafia sold out to the Government, privateers who sailed in the name of the law. His presence brought trouble; but his absence, a war. I don't get into your business, but you kill the competition. Divide and conquer. The analysis of neurons, fighting bacteria against bacteria while my soldiers finish off the survivors. The Corporal Government didn't care what they did, be it cell trafficking, rape, or torture, as long as their power didn't grow too much, as long as they fulfilled the mission they were given.

Diagnosis: colon

-*"Why do you like that part of the body?"*

—Who knows... There are those who are more of the rich, like neurologists; I sympathize with the poor.

It was the corner of the world, a peripheral area, a marginal area. He had some control of resources, and the body did not want a revolt in that area, since the expenses would be in the millions. The bacterial mafia dominated drugs, games and bets, and nothing could be done, they were part of the microbiota. The cells of the colon suffered extortion and blackmail, and life was hard in that place, a jungle where they had to become beasts in order to survive. Hope never came, one dregs after another, some softer than the last, but dregs at last. The absorption of those substances was not the happiest job in the world, and many cells were already beginning to tire.

Diagnosis: cancer

-Why does cancer exist?

—Biology has been created from the struggle. evolution is so just a disagreement with the current system of that environment.

-"I didn't choose to be like that. Why can't we change?

-"So the DNA decided. Don't embarrass your family, the last thing I want is a cancer child. The macrophages would kill you off or you would endanger your body.

- "And why don't I have the opportunities or the resources to other cells? Reply!

-"Enough, I said!" You were born as a colon cell and you will die like this

At that moment his face and his thoughts changed forever. His mother didn't notice it, but his DNA had already mutated, he was already master of his destiny. He clandestinely collected cells from the colon, and the anti-establishment organization began to maneuver. Some members were caught, fell, or reported to the government, but the organization was already consolidated and, as it did not show symptoms that were signs of its growth, it remained under the shadow of the largest intelligence agency: "the health services." The leader did not look like his parents, he was a totally indifferent cell, just like his followers. "They forced us into this, they just wanted equality. If I am a cell of the same body, why don't I have the same rights as the neurons, the resources of the lung, the energy of the myocardium? I will end this inequality, I will destroy this system."

Diagnosis: metastases

Expand yourself, break the horizons of your genetics, travel where you want. Your determination has changed the fate of this body, being you a little cell.

The organ is already taken, but nothing has changed. A simple routine analysis will raise doubts and, if it were to reach higher levels, a simple military operation by the Health Service could undo many years of efforts. We need to seize more organs, make new speeches, rally rebels from other areas to the cause. Time is running out and the bleeding, anemia and weight loss can no longer be hidden. We must take a train by force and distribute ourselves in strategic organs such as the lungs or the bones. Some cells will die along the way, but it is the price to pay, it is for a just cause, for the freedom of my people. We must overthrow the state.

Diagnosis: fever

-*"An eye for an eye, the philosophy that will blind the world."*

-*"Well, we'll all walk with glasses and canes," said the body before the infection.*

-"Burn them all," the general said to his troops, blinded of hate.

-"But General, our men are there..."

-"I have given an order, soldier.

The temperature rose on the battlefield, and the warriors, ready for anything, avenging the death of their fallen comrades, wanted the head of the responsible virus, bacteria or fungus. They cut down their enemies with a sword without a handle, they bombarded war zones regardless of the army or civilians, it was just collateral damage. That was the politics of fever, a boiling revenge, a car bomb where you drive frantically against your target, and that proud body whose thinking borders on madness will continue to do so. Either you die or you die. If I win, you're dead; and if I lose, you're dead, because you won't have anything to eat. You see? In the end I win.

Diagnosis: vaccines

An injury brought him to our center, he had cut his hand. He was treated and tetanus toxoid reactivation was indicated.

The command center was concerned about the new enemy, and the intelligence service was tasked with solving it. A helicopter commanded by the head of Corporal External Intelligence arrived. He wore glasses, synonymous with his intellect and hours of reading; an impeccable suit and an air of determination to do anything for his nation. He took an enemy commander to the headquarters room, with his arms cut off and morale destroyed by countless tortures, and the chief ordered him to speak, to betray his own species, and he had no choice: he told about his formations , its structure, the preferred terrain and its weaknesses. The counteroffensive was carried out successfully and the problem was solved. They imprisoned the commander in a high security memory prison until his testimony is needed again or until he dies in a few years and it is necessary to look for another general.

Diagnosis: myocardial personality

I entered the hospital and, to my luck, found countless students, as varied as their topics of conversation. They radiated different emotions: stress, tiredness, happiness and joy. It was such a shock that I sat down to write.

They were hearts that simply walked among so many lifeless people, some healthy and many broken. They beat! As an order of nature, they were never quiet, they never cared about that picture of atheroma that suffocated them with bad comments. Heart failure, a product of the cruelties of reality, hypertrophied them; the hypertension of failure damaged layers in their trustworthy endothelium, myocarditis of disappointments and more... They just beat ignoring the seriousness of their condition. What did their hearts carry? Dreams, dammit! dreams! They were their hemoglobin in the face of global anemia, and they had enough to fill a blood bank. Some died because they did not have cardiologists, not those who wear a gown, but those who steal moments, draw sighs and leave memories. Cardiologists who had such a sick heart that they learned to treat all kinds of syndromes because they had no choice. And you will see them out there, with their clogged arteries, with sutures from a recent operation, with a myxoma that prevents them from giving their all. And you will see them out there, with a myocardial personality, transporting their dreams until they come true... or die.

Diagnosis: my neuron

A girl, isolated, cried inconsolably for a fact with his partners. I listened to her and the truth is that it was not that bad. I researched about her and came to the conclusion that her classmates they envied her. I don't want to see her like this again. You want to be a neurosurgeon so I wrote something to motivate his passion.

I named it that way, in a unique and irreplaceable way. You had to take care of her; Even the slightest damage would last a lifetime, and those magnificent functions it performs, such as stimulating the release of serotonin, commanding muscles to smile, and promoting dilation in certain blood vessels, could disappear. Being so selective, she was marginalized by the other cells and she felt terrible about it. She was crying, so I went to her side beating like a whole heart. I explained to her that she was not meant to be next to adipose tissues, faneras, and endothelium, that she was for me, to support my functions, to tell me when to speed up or when to stop, to be my partner in this body that some, who don't know of medicine, they call life. She understood how important it was and I kissed her with the force of my ventricles. The years go by while I inspire his Newtonian logic with my blood and the years go by while he balances my wildest arrhythmias.

Diagnosis: anesthesia

I observed an operation, and in the middle of it was a soul that it didn't fit. The patient worsened and that was when she came out, saved his life and returned to his shadow. In the end everyone knew about the surgeon, but not from that unknown girl.

- I asked him: "What are you?"

-He replied: "Anesthesiologist."

He felt nothing in the surgical room of life, excessively anesthetized by the blows, reaching a spiritual standstill. My heart was barely beating. She arrived with the intention of saving me, cardiopulmonary resuscitation of emotions, oxygen of dreams and desire, adrenaline of courage and inspiration. She saved me, she saved me, and I can barely remember. The merits went to the surgeon named "Lucky" and his assistant "Lucky." I looked for her everywhere and, despite being almost imperceptible, I ended up finding her, I thanked her and we started to get to know each other. I was surprised by his humility. She is a hidden hero, working in the darkness of the unconscious, maintaining the complicated balance of the human body when it is most chaotic, and helping without expecting a single "thank you." She only sees the lives she saved, those ignorant souls who don't know they are breathing for her. For an instant I was anesthetized and I loved her, although it was for a moment, but I loved her. I loved his beautiful intelligence, his indeclinable vocation, his infinite humility.

Diagnosis: epithelium

I met a wonderful dermatologist and was surprised that, being the best in the place, she had slightly damaged skin. Despite his age, he radiated life. I asked him why dermatology among so many branches, and he replied that thanks to a friend and he showed me his last letter.

He had beautiful skin. Every cell in her body managed to imitate Aphrodite. Touching her was a pleasure and kissing her, not to mention. Time finally put her to the test, it created scars where there were none, pimples where there was a beautiful face, tears where a smile predominated. I couldn't bear to see her like this, "sad", because in my eyes, she was still beautiful. I invited her to study, and ignoring luck among so many injuries, she discovered her passion.

—Epithelia! -told me-. That is what I want, to heal everyone who has suffered like me, heal their skin, and if I cannot, at least eliminate the sores on their soul, that they understand that they are magnificent with their scars, with their spots and with their keloids.

The art of the skin was his science, and he began to love himself from his epithelium to his deepest organs. She already knows her worth, she shows her body with the pride of thousands of defects and millions of virtues, she does not put on makeup, you see her living experiences with her patients and revolutionizing her field, as she affirms that the best skin cream is happiness.

I invited her to a coffee and we talked like never before: she, about her epithelia; and I, of my hearts. Despite her pimples and scars, she looked more beautiful than when she had her epithelium intact.

Diagnosis: speech therapist

Seeking to clarify doubts about speech therapy, I entered an apartment where, on the walls, many titles and certificates had been hung, although only one caught my attention.

- What a beautiful letter.

—It was the first one I wrote as soon as I was able to communicate, because I also needed a speech therapist.

Hello mother:

You don't know how good it feels to say something. It's been many years without being able to express what I feel. Mother, I laugh at those people who think that the world is ending because they cannot communicate with someone, when I need someone to help me communicate with the world. Mother, you don't know how frustrating it is not being able to say "I love you", "take care", "I miss you", "hug me", imprisoned in the solitude of a voice that refuses to come out. Mother, when I can communicate with you, I will spare no words or frequency, I will tell you everything: my secrets, my mistakes, thank you and I love you. I owe everything to you, your determination to get me to speak, your constant faith, every gesture of encouragement you gave me even when you were crying behind the door, as if you believed it was your fault. You took away many luxuries to pay me for the best treatments. Today

I speak thanks to you, mother, and you know what? A doubt never left my mind: what will become of those who do not have a being like you? I have the obligation to learn to speak, to communicate and to express myself in the best possible way, those beings who need me.

Diagnosis: geriatrician

A soul that decided to say goodbye to others, give them a pleasant time before leaving, because their condition was not the best, although not everyone remembered her, like babies. The extremes tend to be equal, but unlike children, the elderly are not as well liked by their parents.

The culmination of a lifetime ended similar to its beginning, like a lesson that indicated that it should be taken advantage of. They had wrinkles of experience; rebellious gray hair to dyes; eyes, some full of joy, others ignorant of that word. He was a large neonate, a sharp mind in a withered body, the curse of time exposed in human form. They had more pain than smiles, more problems than movements, more emptiness than hope. Broken arteries of disappointment, heart attacks of joy, silent diseases of great surprises. The sphincters forgot their function, memory went for a walk, the view looked well at the soul, but did not see the world. Abandonment and visits, some were worries and others burdens, tears that escaped from the face for one of thousands of reasons. I decided to take care of them; they were the most beautiful thing in the world in the worst of its facets, the autumn of humanity, the target of the worst situations. I saw them and it was like seeing a new universe, some plants and other castles, some books and other ashes, some old people and other children.

Diagnosis: iatrogenic

A child suffering from pain, twenty four hours of diagnosed paralytic ileus and no one had done anything. He asked to die by not taking it anymore; in fact, it was supposed to be. A nurse with a Levin saved him at the last minute.

The stomach went on strike and stopped working; I couldn't continue under those conditions. It all accumulated and the discomfort and painful strains began. He was stuffed and undernourished; it was like a safe where "nothing goes in and nothing comes out". The hours turned into blows; waiting, in torture; and that room, in the basement of an executioner. The ultrasound exposed the culprit, and it was up to the doctors to judge him. These corrupt judges did nothing, corrupted by ignorance or indolence, and the stomach continued to strike. Tears were observed in a tortured child and the helplessness of his parents when they heard: "What have I done to be like this?" The world fell on their shoulders and they had to hold back the tears to give the strength they did not have. His friends came and he could hardly receive them. One of them didn't even want to look at him, he refused to see him like that. An angel came, placed a probe through his nose and expelled all the contents. Then the stomach ended the strike and the trauma remained for life. Years later, the boy became a doctor, and while studying Surgery he was shocked:

what happened was not an accident, but torture; it was not unexpected, but preventable; It wasn't a mistake, it was iatrogenic.

Diagnosis: pathology

I discovered a man who seemed to be with the dead, but his eyes knew how to describe life. We talked and he invited me to his work. We walked in and there were two bodies on the table.

-Do you see? —that man said to me before two bodies open, to which he himself replied:

—One is a young woman, very beautiful; I think she's a bikini model, well, she was. The other is an elderly psychologist who has helped countless people. I have read your books and they are magnificent. Returning to the question, here you can only see what the human being is: a bag of bones, bile, tissues, lipids and the like. Since I started this profession, I have realized that. I stopped liking women and my admiration for the catrinas began.

- "The catrinas?" I asked surprised.

—Yes, the catrinas, those beings that represent death, which is something natural, at least for me. Before choosing my partner, I ask myself if she is a catrina, if I will find her beautiful, despite what "tissue, bile and bones" is. I wonder if, regardless of her form, I will continue to love her, if her soul will remain even after death. I'll tell you something, kid. This young woman has already been overshadowed by another who teaches more, who dresses better or who has more style. However, with the psychologist, very important people have written to me hurt by their loss. They will prepare an admirable burial and their work will be immortalized.

-"Have they written to you?"

—Yes, well, he was my lover, or rather, my catrina.

Diagnosis: diagnosis

Why are they so wrong? With how easy it is to say this disease is such, and it is treated with this and that's it. Piece of cake," said the most ignorant patient I know.

Meanwhile, what can it be? Too many things influence, such as age, epidemiology or race. What has your body suffered? What illness will he have inherited from his family? He presents signs and refers symptoms of at least seven diseases with totally different treatments and variable prognoses. Let's do tests to rule it out, let's look at his blood, his chest, his urine, his feces. Tell me how acidic your body is, I want to know even the amount of potassium you have. We think we know what it is, but we have three patients with the same disease defending the theory of individuality: "There are no diseases, only sick." If we manage to eliminate all suspicions and still find nothing, we are left with discard diseases, those people who are at the end of your contact list. In case we find nothing to explain such a situation, we are left with a word that hides our "idiopathic" ignorance.

Diagnosis: medical ethics

"Have medical ethics," a patient told me after disrespecting me and I responded as she deserved.

I have sacrificed too much for the human race, for the well-being of my species. I carry the knowledge of your body, of your life and of your death. Many times you are more my priority than your family's. Your health, in one way or another, speaks of me and my treatment. I am willing to sacrifice hours in surgery to save you, develop my ingenuity to discover your pathology, fight against my superiors to prioritize your case... but there is something you should know, dear patient: if you think I should not eat or sleep to care for you without being an urgency, for the simple fact that you think you are special, you forget that I believe it more, because your life depends on me. If you offend me and expect me to do nothing to be a doctor, you forget that I have a pride forged by teachers who did not trust my ability and I shut their mouths. If you hit me, expect a fist to your face developed from practicing hundreds of maneuvers that will save your life. If your problems frustrate you and you expel them with me, you forget that I have my own added to all those who visit me; expect a more violent response. Don't confuse kindness with weakness, dedication with slavery, being peaceful with being crippled.

Diagnosis: profession

I met a doctor who worked with a passion like no other. He was an overwhelming learner and his curiosity was insatiable. I met him; his past was full of shortcomings and his profession frustrated.

"I had no choice but to leave," were his last words. mixed with helplessness and hate.

I got tired and left, sick of prescribing pills that my patients couldn't get, of performing Paleolithic procedures, of using products in poor condition. It hurt me to see my patients worsen due to lack or theft of the antibiotic that would save them, of the antihypertensive that would prevent that stroke, of the insulin that would control their diabetes. Shortage of gloves to operate; three instead of six, you had to round up. Poor hygiene, violation of parameters, act in those conditions or let them die. It looked like war in full peace, a camp in the center of a city. Meetings that didn't resolve anything, lost study time, years, theses, doctorates, diplomas... For what? If you can't work, if you can't even live. Sad reality of the one who saves lives, exploited by his superiors, demanded by his patients. Free is not usually valued. "Without life for medicine, without money for medicine, without practicing medicine well." The equation was a mockery of health and those who profess it. White was not so white, dreams were not fulfilled, difficulties lashed, and the same hope told me: "You have no choice but to leave."

Diagnosis: nurses

—How well you get along with your nurses…

—Obviously, they are a very important pillar.

"We need your support," said the one with years of experience in his profession. Your hands, your skills, your knowledge and your disposition are essential. There is talk of hierarchy, but I do not consider them soldiers under the command of doctors, but the co-pilot of a plane that, instead of traveling to Paris, decided to cross the Bermuda Triangle. It's the laughs that lift you up, the shoulders where you rest, the eyes you trust and the witness that saves you. They carry a great responsibility and very practical virtues. Don't confuse his loyalty with submission; There is no worse enemy than a great ally. You will know hell when you are missing and peace of mind in their company. We are not so different, professions that kiss the human species, that yearn for its salvation by watching it die. Appreciate them, they are a white rose spotted with red in a black sea.

Diagnosis: faith

An incredible man, as a person and as a doctor, who was around the room, diagnosing and professing inspiration in his patients.

—I believe in God and, although not everyone believes in him, they do believe in something higher, some faith. I find that faith and make them live by it. Not only of bread the man lives. Human beings need to believe in something to live," said a doctor whose survival rate for his patients was incredible. He presented a synchronous duality in his being: extremely logical in medicine and an ancient Greek priest with his patients. Exact in quantities with the doses and a prophet regarding his dreams. Get out of here and find your unicorn! The philosophy that allowed a spoiled girl to comply with the treatment.

"If your wife were alive, she would still love the man you've become,"- he told an inveterate lover who fell into bed after becoming a widower. They talked about her for days and the evolution was masterful. I saw him convince a sixty-eight-year-old man to try out to be an astronaut if he recovered from his accident.

"Why are you cheating on them?"- they asked him once.

—I believe in an invisible being who can with everything, in a fight against a fallen angel who wants to torture us for eternity, and like me, millions believe in this. Others believe in Allah, in Shiva, in fascism, in communism and in their mothers. They believe in impossible dreams and fight for them. What did Da Vinci believe in to create so many works or Michelangelo his paintings? Did Jules Verne lie to us all with his writings? Man needs to believe in something to live. And how, knowing this, the doctors, knowing that the human needs something that fills his soul, that forces him to get out of bed, do they not use it? How dare you tell me that if they keep the dead alive like vegetables by means of apparatus? I place faith in a living body that has lost its soul, whatever it is.

Diagnosis: polytrauma

Death was bored and the worst happened: a spontaneous cave-in and lives lost without warning. Terror set in in seconds and humanity began to shine. help became in compass of that scenario. Politics and religion were forgotten to start fighting as a species, to fight as humans.

The hospital mobilized the elite. Meeting of specialties, intelligence sprouted from the guard corps. The worst thing you've imagined we saw, the worst thing you've ever seen we had to cure. The organization sat on its throne. Keeping calm in that chaos was audacity. Injuries, personnel, materials, stretchers, blood... Not even the biggest painting could capture such a moment. Some mild and others to the operating room, some screaming and others unconscious. Operate and be saved, operate and die. There was no time for tears or for celebration. Kill the feelings and continue your work. For us they are not figures. We got to know them, we were by their side in their worst facet, we discovered their past, we diagnosed their luck and we fought for their future. Some of us even knew his name, his age, and even his blood. The hours already hurt, hunger increased, hygiene evaporated. "As if that mattered, they need me," was the prevailing voice that rose from the unconscious. The relay arrived and I didn't want to leave, as if everything I had done was not enough, as if I had some fault for what happened. The patient arrives with the traumas in the body and we keep them in the soul.

Diagnosis: bioanalyst

I entered the laboratory and was surprised that even on his birthday he was working. I looked at her with a "what are you doing here?" face.

"They need me," answered that beautiful girl with glasses. looking at his microscope.

—We all need you, both your patients and your doctors, but today is your birthday.

—It's not that bad; It's just another year.

It's another year for that girl with microscopic details, with glasses full of knowledge, with a smile full of life.

One more year for those who seek the priceless, explorer of the essential, heels of elegance and tenderness.

One more year for the only person who will discover your emotional anemia, if you cannot heal the wounds or if your self-esteem has leukopenia. He hugs you and you forget the world, he talks to you and you go into a trance, he kisses you and you lose your senses.

One more year for that bioanalyst who knows the bacteria of hate, pain and sadness. It became the antibiogram of my life.

One more year for those who cultivate experiences. A few minutes by your side they will create millions of memories.

And I know that he will continue to say: "It's not a big deal, it's just another year for that wonderful woman, that impeccable scientist, my laboratory of emotions."

Diagnosis: psychiatry

A madman in a straitjacket in the mental hospital. They had entered it recently. According to the doctors, he was the sanest madman in the center, but there was too much freedom in that person. Her day was spent reading, exercising, meditating, and writing.

-What is life and how can I live it to the fullest? I want to do what I love and get paid for it. Why should I settle for something that brings me profit but that I don't like? I want to travel through the feelings of the world. If it's going to hurt, make it so bad that I faint. If I'm going to cry, don't let a single tear remain inside me. If I'm going to laugh, my cheeks hurt. I want to find someone who makes me forget the rest so that I can, once and for all, enjoy that treasure, to focus on someone who really matters. I want to speak without reservations or prejudices, that my opinion is the law of my world, that my conscience guides my destiny. Praise the beautiful, both an incomprehensible work of art and a fascinating woman, not out of lust and interest, but for the pleasure of it. Heal souls and bodies, be part of the fulfillment of the best plans. Align once and for all my chaotic thoughts, my unbreakable soul and my disastrous body. Having so much in my account to be able to buy what the rich can't reach. Enjoy the knowledge, not only from books, but also from people, loneliness, the nature of silence and the noise of technology. Save in the city to walk through the fields, and in those fields, discover how to earn in the city. Bathing in the rain, getting lost in the sea, climbing and finding God while passing out from exhaustion or starvation. Always carry a sheet that reminds me that my life was not insignificant, in which I wrote down the best of it. I want to surround myself with crazy, misunderstood, lonely. Such complex universes in the middle of the streets. I want to wear rags and still know my worth, wear suits and not have my ego soar. I want to do what I want at the time I want. I want to achieve such freedom.

—And why don't you go find what you want?

Diagnosis: chronic

"Human beings are a damned madman who crawls into the abyss in a way as slow as imperceptible", said that philosopher of thousand diseases, almost all produced by himself.

- "Damned conscience, it ruins everything with its desire to die, with its self-hatred,"-said the unconscious with its hard work twenty-four hours every day during life.

-Why you smoke? Leave drugs, exercise and protect yourself when having sex. Avoid traumas with your follies. Do you think it is easy to weld bones that are often dysfunctional, eliminate hundreds of toxins from the lungs, push hypertension out of the door, clean the grease from your arteries after sucking your fingers and have to live with incurable beings in your genitals? My works are as countless as your whims. The chronic makes fun of you, it puts you to sleep with its arguments. I am the butler, and you, the naughty boy. You are the debtor and I am the family that supports you... The problem is that we live in the same body.

He opened a bottle to forget everything for a moment and the unconscious realized something: «I suppose that our desire to destroy is impregnated in the DNA, including us in that list. Chronic suicide is a treat for this breed."

Diagnosis: ophthalmologist

A girl left her assistantship for overly demanding teachers, by teachers who had forgotten that they were ever students.

Women who barely saw, had frustrated their desire, and I looked at them, hurt by how they trampled on their dreams. She wanted to cure the eyes, and for me she was perfect in that task. She, whose soul was transparent like crystal clear, made your eyes dilate when you heard her name, her light caused miosis. My fovea took her job seriously so as not to forget the smallest detail when I enjoyed her company. It does not have a single form, its iris is of many colors. In an afternoon by his side, humor reigns supreme and can make you blink several times to confirm if it's real. He's good at leaving your mind like the sclera, and he knows how to mess with your optic nerve. And, even so, he wants to leave him because of the opinion of some women who barely see, because of the opinion of some women who did not take a deep look at their soul.

Diagnosis: stress

The test was only a few days away and we were all nervous. How is it possible that a simple sheet full of questions can put a human being accustomed to this ritual of development like this?

—The tests are coming; I guess I'll have to get dressed -said stress.

A thin-looking being with obvious baldness and a scared smile put on his tie. He suffered from gastritis. If you looked closely, you would discover the canker sores in his mouth. His face conveyed insecurity, insomnia had tattooed dark circles under his eyes and frustration had dented his body. He sat next to all the students, watching what was happening. Some very strong recited the content in his face with indifference; others forgot much of it. He was restless by nature. I was always sweating or had bad digestion. It is said that he was strong, a complex of skill and dexterity, a multiplier of qualities. His abuse would result in disaster; overdoses would finish him off. Beep-beep. The alarm goes off, he gets up, sees the message —a medicine test— and is filled with energy, because they brightened his morning.

-"It's payback time for using me so much."

Diagnosis: curettage

I don't know his reasons, but he was in the curettage room. They had to repeat it, because there were remains. I was too scared for experience, and asked me to warn about it.

 The doctor put the bandages on his eyes and began to work. Blind procedure they called it. The mind was filled with images and thoughts, regret was crowned, the risks began to multiply.

—I curse sex, abortion, hormones and bleeding. You have me here. Fear embraces me while the doctor explains that we must repeat it. There were still remains. What will become of that soul that they are murdering? -I wonder.

-"It's not a soul. It hasn't formed yet. -Is the answer that they always give me

For me it is, it is part of me since I was a cell. Guilt kills me for it and karma comes to mock. My uterus claims me and judges me, and I don't know what explanation to give it. My whole body hates me and despises me, and I don't know how to escape from my own skin, how to convince a jury to whom I cannot lie, a jury full of evidence that wants to see me imprisoned in the jail of madness, of my innocence. .

Diagnosis: social case

A man was brought to the hospital, as he was in the street screaming from pain. No relative came with him; He was transferred by officers.

The pains suffer alone. My family had abandoned me and I barely remembered the language. They bumped into me without realizing it and my hip started to complain. Nobody helped me. Will they know I'm human? I closed my eyes and opened them in a hospital, tied up like an animal, penetrated with drips and needles. The doctors began to speak and I could barely understand them: "He is fit to operate" was the only thing that managed to capture my mind. My body reacted on its own and the nurse gave me a painkiller too roughly. The pain brought me out of sleep and the stitches reaffirmed the operation. An experiment for them, with no one to claim me. How I miss my family! I don't remember how I ended up like this, how I became a social case. Bear with me, doctor. You are the only thing I have left.

Diagnosis: inhuman

He heard screams from a person who was supposedly being healed. One of the chief surgeons, outraged by that act, went to check. The resident had not used any anesthetic, the doctor ended up angry and the patient in pain.

"It is not a piece of meat that is on this table, it is a person", that being with intelligence for cuts and sutures always told us, with more energy than many young people, with more heart than many old people. If I break it is to fix, if damage is to heal; My goal is to see you better. No disgust for blood, skin or pus, with all care not to hurt yourself. He's cold enough to do his job, human enough to understand your fear. How difficult is the role of that executioner who tortures without desire! Scrape the dead and pain is born, synonymy of life, if the tissue hurts it is good. Being that gives you the confidence to close your eyes and not know if you will open them. Your future lies in his hands, what a burden that man's! How many will he have saved? How many did he disappoint? Even so, he continues to smile, determined to carry that weight on his back.

—Those who make a patient scream fail! —That action was inconceivable, that naked, vulnerable, wounded being. He has given you the opportunity to heal him, to teach you, with the certainty that everything you will do will be magnificent. Never disappoint that soul that already suffers, that comes desperate to you, that feels, loves and cries. Treat her like the human being she is, treat her like you are in her position.

Diagnosis: pregnancy

A pregnant woman visited the office complaining about her symptoms, typical of pregnancy, but at the same time, she was very happy to have that creature gestating inside her. I couldn't understand her.

The price of life is a bit ironic, cravings cannot always be satisfied, you will not always be able to taste a good meal without being interrupted by vomiting. Sometimes you are fine and other times diabetes surprises you with its sweets and hypertension plays with your emotions. The column bothers you and the knees complain of your weight; the charge they carry is double. Infections take advantage and care is doubled. Kicks make you happy and the slightest circumstance gets on your nerves. The curve you always wanted is on the wrong side and the beauty you never had is presented in an artistic way. Goddess of the kingdom, dresses are your new fashion, questions are the usual. What does sex matter if you want it just the same? What does time matter if they are usually born when they please? Hormones are in dispute and temperament varies. In a few hours you are sad, happy, melancholic and furious. What a beautiful spectacle! You, in chaos for meaningless things; me, trying to understand the incomprehensible. Proud of her suffering, happy of her figure, two

lives and two souls with so much to go through, with so much to
live.

Diagnosis: fetus

I was in the dining room when I noticed that he was sitting next to me. one of the most eminent doctors in the hospital. His robe was impeccable and his face described knowledge. He had an air of controlled superiority. He did not have to be there, it is as if a president had lunch in a humble home.

-"Tell me your story," I said to that icon of medicine.

—I love ontogeny; based on it I created my life.

Before I went out into the world, I asked myself what I wanted and put the plan into my DNA. Every minute detail was in it. It took time, I don't deny it. Having thought of everything, only action remained, and I began my career as an ovum for three hours a day fighting for my dreams. Graduated, I became a blastocyst. I was already in the right place, so I started to grow and created a placenta that included the will, determination and guts to communicate with my mother, that person who has lived longer than me and who provided me with what I needed for my development. Transformed into an embryo, the world already knew about me, although I was not very pleasant in the eyes of everyone. I had to manage to continue growing, training. I have to say that my mother's words of encouragement helped me a lot at that stage. She was glad every time he kicked, as if to say "I'm

51

here." The time came when I could go out into the world perfectly, even with stumbling blocks and a little immature, but I could go out. I decided to wait, as there was a risk of premature death and the change would be very abrupt. I kept preparing. My movements were stronger, almost painful, and my mother could barely contain me. I decided to go out, my water broke and I traveled through that tunnel that I did not know where it would take me. At birth, I cried, and it was so loud that humans ran to see me. The world recognized me and welcomed me into its arms.

-"And why do you have supper with ovules like us?"

-"So I don't forget who I am."

—Was it three hours a day dedicated to your future?

-Minimum. My dreams could not die from starvation.

Diagnosis: childbirth

A pregnant woman was talking to us about how excited she was to have a child. It was already almost nine months; the hour was drawing near.

Life gave a scream and the contractions began. The water ran out of his legs; there was little left for the arrival. The vagina began to dilate and the pain became overwhelming, to such an extent that she questioned having come to this. The contractions were too much for the muscles and the baby was already wanting to come out. In the delivery room, forced to push almost forcefully, it was an echo in her subconscious. Push, Push! It was very easy to say, but torture to do. Shouting was a luxury, because one had to save strength. Whoosh! A cut in the vagina. Whoosh! The fetus must be helped. The head could already be seen, the image was as beautiful as it was traumatic, a light in the midst of that chaos. He quickly left that humid environment and cried as a pathognomonic sign of being alive. The mother was happy, but it was not finished yet: the tears had to be sutured, the stitches sewn in the vagina, the damage repaired, and the trauma reconstructed. When she had her baby in her arms, the world stopped and she forgot about pain. It's amazing that women go through that; It's amazing that some sons don't value their mothers.

Diagnosis: neonate

I found my old neonatology professor. What a relentless woman! The inmates feared him, as well as fatigue: With her you did not stop working or learning. A dictatorship based in discipline and knowledge.

She is a mother of more than a million children. He never sees them grow up, but still, he keeps them alive until the moment they leave the hospital. He watches them in the school incubator, he usually examines them daily; Let's say you perform a physical examination of the soul. Find cephalohematomas full of doubts; toxic erythema to those allergic to suspend; macrosomic and microsomic, some for being arrogant and others for being ignorant. She just reassures them and keeps a close eye on them. You know that some newborns go through that physiological stage. She is an expert in her field, confident exchange transfusion when close to kernicterus, when close to throwing in the towel, disciplinary surfactant to each hyaline membrane of laziness, immobilization and rest to each personal fracture, physiotherapy and support to each paralysis.

¿Why am I going to lie to you? I hate her and I love her, she tires me and inspires me, she scolds me and pampers me. It was one of my mothers, because she kept me alive until the moment I left the hospital.

Diagnosis: greed

While writing a medical history, I became aware of a man whose family was more concerned with his fortune than with him. They paid more attention to the lawyer than to the patient. I looked at him, and his eyes were so expressive that I had to write what they said.

Gold was his companion, but health deserted him. She says that he ignored her for that sin. Surrounded by the best doctors, nurses and technologies, it was as if Midas himself had fallen ill. How will you eat delicacies if you cannot use your mouth? Who will you impress with your outfits if you can't leave the room? How could you cure gold? His position was so rich and his situation so poor, his family was his property and they claimed it. More questions to the lawyer than to the doctor, more attention to the will than to the treatment. Health personnel surprised to hear "when will he die?" instead of "does he have salvation?"

I looked at him perplexed and apparently he understood my question. HE he replied to himself:

"Rich and poor, surrounded by many and only the truth, with modern cars and in a wheelchair, cared for by strangers and abandoned by my relatives, with a mansion and a sad room, with millions in the bank and bankrupt my life".

Diagnosis: anger

—Two bodies lying on the ground: one, severely tortured; and another, shot in the head. Most likely the killer committed suicide. One of the things that my career has taught me is to control my anger -was what that forensic doctor said at the conference by way of reflection.

"Kill, break, and smash!" Have no mercy! —he says to the mind as he blinds it with the scarf of hate. Do not let reasons, the order is not for you, but for your body. It has no fixed shape: one day it is a knife; another, a mallet; another, some hands. Walk through the city transforming realities, boil the blood to change passion to crime. Cold revenge sits waiting for her, abusers use her as an argument, and those who assault, to fill their void. It is the fire that burns everything and at the same time devours you. He doesn't want death, he enjoys it. He sits at the table to serve bruises from beatings with caused fractures, he adores the symphony of torture, the screams of horror, and he loves not knowing how to differentiate between fear and anxiety that reigns before suicide. It never dies, it goes from soul to soul, from being to being. She's cunning. He chose an Achilles heel almost impossible for human beings to achieve: forgiveness.

-"Kill, break, and smash!" Have no mercy! says anger from the Colosseum, while humans die in the arena.

Diagnosis: gluttony

An obese teenager was fighting for his life in therapy: diabetic ketoacidosis was his urgency. The grandmother was unaware of her pathological condition. Apparently they lived alone; maybe grandma induced him a lifelong disease to his beloved grandson.

Eat to be strong! The motto of a thousand tons. His weapon is the flavor that hides the garbage, the sausage-shaped gristle, the sugar in sodas, the fat in hamburgers. Love excesses and banquets, flaccid and lipid. Her dogs, Obesity, Gout, and Diabetes, follow her around as a show of loyalty, and she obliges them with countless humans. Hates the stomach; that is why it makes him suffer so much, regardless of the torture, having emesis or bad digestion. Refill it until you can't anymore. The pancreas surrenders and that is when it considers itself victorious. Thirty years maximum left. He uses love as an excuse to delve into the new generations, beings who have neither knowledge nor guilt. He doesn't want the food, he wants the dessert; he doesn't want milk, he wants cola; he's not fat, he's cute! Gluttony mocks humans for falling for such arguments. Cholesterol and glucose are your preferred values, your effectiveness ratio, your wealth ratio. He hired advertising so that there is a McDonald's on every corner with the phrase: "Raise your hands and open your mouths! This is a robbery!".

Diagnosis: envy

Walking through the park, I noticed a woman looking at her camera. It seemed that she missed him even holding her in her hands, it seemed that she was part of her life. I got closer and noticed that on his face he had the mark of a butterfly so characteristic of lupus, I introduced myself and we started talking.

His entire life was in front of the camera; her face received more care and attention than many children; modeling was her passion; and seduction, his game. He knew of the envy that he provoked among his companions, but he never expected a betrayal from his own body. His body got tired of the makeup, the treatments and the excesses to which he was subjected. Her defenses attacked her and her face flew out of the magazines, never to return. He couldn't exercise because of the pain in his joints. Rebellious nodes to treatment, they wanted to stand out as much as she did. She stopped being that brilliant woman for an anemic and tired one. The mark of lupus will haunt her forever as a reminder of the danger of envy, as a warning not to trust even her own body.

Diagnosis: lust

Concern on a face that was waiting for serology. "Positive" said that paper, as if it were a list of the grim reaper and his name were indelible letters. He saw in him something more than death, loneliness, since AIDS was already in his body.

She put on her most erotic clothes and put on makeup so that no one would recognize her. Before leaving, he kept AIDS and other diseases in his bag. He liked going out with company, transmitting his fragrance, his stench of misfortune. Lust left the room looking to ruin souls. A fly landed on the cloth and took her to the red room with her best lingerie. Handcuffs, chains, dildos and more. They played with them; He had fun like never before with that subject prey to pleasure. She, transmitting death in her fluids. It ended, and the subject left happy and unaware of his condition. He would no longer be tied to the bed, but to lifelong treatments; I would no longer leave the red room, I would be trapped by thousands of prejudices; He would no longer be a trustworthy person, as he became a sea of disappointments. And lust continues to come out every night with her wallet, with her fluids, with her illnesses but without her face, ruining lives with pleasure, entering rooms that will remain empty.

Diagnosis: sloth

A car accident. Almost the entire family died, except for one man, the oldest of all. When he came to, the information was withheld from him, but it didn't take long for him to realize it. His heart could not stand the reality and after a few days the doctors could not rescue him from unemployment.

The whole body surrendered, decided to rest, lost its why. The brain did not want to think, he left the presidency, he went into retirement. The heart, that tireless organ, stopped. Life hit him where he was weak, literally destroyed him. The mouth did not want to open, the meals would never taste the same, the dinners would not be the same. The eyes closed. He couldn't conceive of a world without familiar faces, he didn't want to see his greatest achievements buried. The legs refused to move. No one would expect him, and he no longer belonged anywhere. He didn't need the strength of his arms to carry his grandchildren, hug his daughter, caress his wife. Laziness proclaimed itself queen, prohibited movement, forgot the desire, burned the whys, changed doing for sleeping, fighting for surrender, will for indifference. Life seemed too hard to him; that is why he intensely sought death.

Diagnosis: pride

A woman in a wheelchair, with more energy than many young people, drew too much attention, I don't know if because of her wild elegance or for not having breasts or hair. I wanted to give a lecture in the oncology ward dedicated to women with breast cancer. I was surprised to read the title of the conference, because it was the worst of the sins.

He stood in the middle of all those women, with the air of a leader who creates others, with all the certainty that his words would change their lives.

—You will be bald, so forget the beauty of your hairstyle. They will cut off your breasts, so you will no longer have what provided food and served for sexuality. You will lose weight, desire and dreams. The world, men and your family will no longer see you as the woman you used to be. Now you're a pitiful, lifeless being who exists to take pills and receive drips.

That room was shocked. The coldness and indifference of his words had no equal. Wasn't she in the same situation?

-"Were they bred for that?" Did they come into the world to leave like that? Have they forgotten who they were and what they fight for? Is it a reason to give up? -He uttered those words in such a way that we didn't know if he was a detective asking questions or a

61

girl who didn't understand anything. He swallowed and spoke as if he had millions to convince.

-"No!" We are women, we were the ones who condemned this world by biting the apple. We, who endured years of differences and managed to be respected, are the backbone of a home, the example for our children and the reason for our men. Indirect authors of poems, photos, paintings and writings. Muses of life, even with little hair and no breasts, we do not stop being goddesses, immortal with our autumnal beauty. Never forget what you are! Women! They endured deliveries, they brought lives, their resistance is enviable. Never stain that word! WOMEN! For his family, for his loved ones, for the world, for the life that, although it mistreated us in the end, will not be able to bring us to our knees. He will never be able to break us. At that moment, she had a coughing fit that forced her to stop. We all worried, but he instantly pulled himself together.

—Be proud, may your last actions be a hug, may your last caresses be a kiss, may your last words change lives.

Diagnosis: microscopic rebellion

I knew an oncologist who was very passionate about cancer prevention. He was an excellent surgeon, but he said that in matters of rebellion it was better to prevent them than to eliminate them. I did not understand him, so which he explained to me.

The strict order of the DNA was broken and a rebellion began against the perfect dictatorship of the body. Incessantly multiplying rebels willing to do whatever it takes to overthrow the omnipotent regime. "Below!" was his motto. It didn't matter how many were subdued. Sometimes the most faithful cell ended up joining the rebellion against the system. He sacrificed breasts while children needed food, wombs to those who wanted to bring life, lungs to those who were inspired, brains full of ideas. Countless organs of power were overthrown. Each government was different: some with vices and diseases; others healthy and reckless. Death cared little. He played dice with them like it was nothing, drained the life out of them and everyone around them. Every time they died, I could see her by my side, carrying their souls saying the same phrase: "Another rebellion that succeeds."

Diagnosis: type 1 diabetes mellitus

*A child in an endocrinology consultation sees a man who turns
face so as not to see the needle that draws blood. This one asks to
the mother: "*

*-Why do they do that?" If they inject you is the most normal thing
world.*

To which the mother responds holding back tears:

-"Not everyone is as strong as you.

She is the bully of children, the pedophile of diseases, the one who
manipulates them with sweets. Life is insulin, death is any
moment. Needles for snacks, three a day. It doesn't even hurt
anymore, or they've already resigned. "Careful!" is the word they
hear the most, both when playing and eating. Careful! It is the echo
of his existence. Sudden fainting visits them and they don't know if
when they open their eyes they will be in another place. How sad is
the irony of filling, constant thirst, constant urination, constant
hunger, skinny as always. The wounds are not weeks, they are
months; and the second house is not the school, it is the hospital.
The cramps do not subside, the fatigue does not go away, the
anxiety appears. They don't bring snacks, they bring syringes; they
are not messy, they follow a strict regulation; They are not
children, they are heroes.

Diagnosis: Legg-Calvé-Perthes syndrome

A man, who was undergoing evolutionary imaging studies to see his condition, his parents tried to give him the happiest childhood they could, since he had a curse on his hip.

A capricious body that, from time to time, left the femur without food. It is said to be the largest, so it could hold up. That frequent whim began to cause discomfort. Blood torture, prolonged fasting began to leave sequelae. What was the child to know of this? He only noticed that his movements were not the same, that his hip did not meet his expectations.

-"We have to take him to the operating room," -said the orthopedist with sadness and hope.

¿That age had? No more than eight, and he already had to be operated, while others visited hospitals for trivial issues; he had to be immobilized, while others ran in their recreations; he had to remain in a wheelchair, while others learned the laws of socializing and making friends. He was imprisoned in a chair inside a house, looking through the window at the freedom of his companions. Over time, he was able to walk and he was a different person, he smiled differently, he lived and breathed with a new frequency and, even so, he was afraid that it would happen again. "Walk!" he said to himself. "Take deep steps, follow your route and not others, take

65

adventurous shortcuts, visit the ones you love, run until you drop, tomorrow you can be in your chair... but today your legs support you."

Diagnosis: bronchial asthma

The lack of air forced him to periodically spray himself. He had certain limitations compared to other children. He was terrified of cold nights, as it announced his arrival.

That was a relentless woman, covered in night. The air lifted her dress showing her white legs as cold as snow. In his mouth he carried the sign of death and suffocation. He kissed without distinction, man or woman, child or old man; his lust had no limits, to such an extent that he never protected himself and left his genetic mark imprinted on his lungs. With his harp he played symphonies for prepared ears, with his lips he stole the air and compressed the chest. He liked blue, cyanosis blue, and he adored the markings on the body called tirajes. The weather changes marked his appointment and he was never late. Sometimes she was jilted by Miss Salbutamol or the Corticoid Queen, but she didn't mind, she had her whole life to see him.

Diagnosis: Down syndrome

Noble family of perfect genetics. Much was expected from that delivery. High-ranking doctors, respected by their peers and loved for their patients. Everything should be fine, but...

Genetics looked to the side and made the mistake: three instead of two; she wanted to be generous, she wanted to give a little more. The world fell on top of those parents with thousands of plans and projects for their little one. They had already prepared even which university he would go to. It was a mockery of his intelligence, a misspelling of fate. What will we do now? How can we repair it? The bottle was emptied, the grass caught fire, and nothing, those owners of life and death could not handle such a scenario. They looked at him with pain, knowing that he would never understand many things, that he would be treated differently, that he would suffer illnesses due to his condition.

There were not many options: abandon it or have the "mistake" of those perfectionists. They decided to love him... They couldn't stop saving a life, much less one created by them. After all, he was his son. They gave her everything and enjoyed that magnificent process of motherhood. That child was truly unique. Still, deep down it wasn't entirely true. The mother sometimes took drugs imagining a different world and the father drank to stay sane. Fate and genetics watched what happened to give three where there should be two.

Diagnosis: alexithymia

An autistic man, too intelligent, had a coefficient which was on par with his coldness. There was something he was unaware of and he set out by all means to find it.

Feelings? FEELINGS. I could tell you the concept of the dictionary, I've learned it perfectly, but to be honest, I don't know, or maybe I can't express it. I know the story of the red thread, but how can I tell a woman that I love her? My thread may be grey. When my family hugs or kisses me, it's not much different than a handshake from a stranger. Affection is an enigma to me. Sad, happy, frustrated or excited; They are just words written in a language that I cannot feel, that my soul has not learned to read. How could you explain to me? I am a winter soldier in a war that he cannot understand, living in subhuman conditions, knowing the sun from books and not from its rays. The emotional fauna is extinct, the view is a snowstorm dressed in white. I, firm in my fort, with the weapon in the hand, I observe how a human approaches. I don't know if he's friend or foe, I don't know whether to let him live or pull the trigger. After all, I'm in a war... that I still don't understand.

Diagnosis: Crohn's disease

*-"Why don't you write about my friend?" I'm sure that something
like that will make her feel good.*

-I only write about diseases.

-"Here's one for you.

Reality began to think: "What if I create a disease to screw up the
lives of humans?" So he called a trained team: Genetics, the
Environment and the Logical brothers —Inmu and Micro—, and
left them the task. The copyright was taken by another, but that
mattered little to reality, since it was adapted to injustices; she
wanted to see her bearers. He found a woman who changed his
perspective, a nymph in a truly dirty game. The canker sores didn't
stop him from talking, much less from laughing. Her digestion
betrayed her with sudden pain, but I never saw a tear or a dent in
her pride. It is said that fever and decay are normal, but she was
hot in a thousand ways and her energy flowed from her delicious
body. Anemia and vomiting, always with her dark skin and the
sexy silhouette of her body; she changed the rules. The treatment
was a sword of broken glass. Having it in your hands for a long
time was torture. Reality stared at her in astonishment. How could
she dance so free, be so spontaneous, amuse beauty and seduce the
masses? Fate asked me: "Why are you writing to her if you don't

71

even know her?" I replied: "I like those oasis people who, in the middle of this desert, are a drink of courage, of resistance. They are the reason to live against the worst odds.

Diagnosis: autistic

That mother had taken her son to many consultations looking for a cure for his isolation and his lack of social understanding. According to her, this was number eleven and she hardly saw any progress.

Why mom? Why so much effort to join the society? A group of people lying to each other, wanting to know about everyone's life except their own. Hypocrites who envy your successes and rejoice at your falls. They have no flaws according to them, but not even Sherlock has found so many in others. I don't want to fall well; I want to be myself. I feel like never in my world, being honest with myself, being at peace with my soul. I can concentrate on tasks that you see as almost impossible. I see many things that they ignore as illogical. I move in a universe that does not want to know anything about the irrational and unheard of society. leave me mom I can help humanity more by creating some invention that you missed by answering a "hello", by checking your social networks. I am a microscope in my laboratory looking for a cure, destined to perform a task as arduous as it is rewarding. I love you, because I know you do it for my good and I will do what I can to make you proud, but you must know that this is my opinion, even if I can't tell you in person, even if it never leaves my lips.

Diagnosis: dengue

The cyclone devastated, increasing the areas where the water accumulated. After a few weeks, the cases of fever and decay arrived. Suddenly, there were too many insects in the environment.

A theater of buzzing, an unparalleled work of mosquitoes Aedes. His audience had peculiar stains, a taste of metal, exhausted from his scene. The greatness of the liver was appreciated when the crown was placed, the exaltation of blood through the mucous membranes. Vomiting queued up and the abdomen screamed during the opera. Muscles and bones ached from clapping so much, and eyes were afraid to go out the door. They said that behind her there was pain. The head could not understand everything and began to ache. As it was forbidden to get up from the seat, the public couldn't wait to go to the bathroom. The symphony of the picada continued to play, an epidemic sonnet, the record that we usually listen to in the living room.

Diagnosis: tetraplegia

He was writing his medical history, and when I started talking with her, she marked my life with indelible ink.

-Hello how are you today? -I was struck by the beauty under those sheets

—And if today I ask you? he told me, to which I went impossible to deny

-"Where have you gone today?" I miss stepping on the sand so much. What have you seen that has left you speechless? If I want to see something, I have two options: search on my mobile or close my eyes, and in both cases it is never the same. Did you hug who you love? I can't, and I have to be unequal with those who do it with me. Did you ask him if he likes you? You know what I mean, don't you? Well, I didn't do it, and I think it's the biggest foolish thing of my life. Maybe he would be here with me or maybe my conscience would be easier, who knows? What does sex taste like? I have guarded my virginity so long that I have turned it into buried treasure. My life is already ruined in a certain way, but you, you have a future, so... tell me about the death of your dreams and the life of your fears, tell me about your most certain doubts, tell me something really sad, let's see if I can succeed smile," -he told me with the fervor of ecstasy.

-"Come see me when you can, doctor." Generally, it is the dead who teach the living to live.

Diagnosis: depression

From time to time she fell into such a deplorable state that it was impossible to imagine that this smiling woman would have to go to the psychologist so many times.

What reason is life, the nonsense of reality, the future that never comes? I don't see the light. According to the doctors, from a bandage that I put on too tight myself. What good is effort if corruption reigns, if beauty has devoured skill? You laugh only to make your muscles work, to trick yourself with dopamine. If you come to understand this cruel world, you will not stop being sad to think about the atrocities of the human being. The inspiration separated from me and the judge gave him all the goods, the desire betrayed me and the energy mocked my face. Trapped in the box of my mind, looking for a key that may not even exist, blindly and hungry, with time running out.

Diagnosis: suicide

A father arrived at the ER with his daughter, who had taken a whole bottle of pills. She was a woman who, according to many, had no reason to.

A peerless woman threatened fate with a knife in her hand. His purpose was admirable; his character, weak. I wanted to write, heal and inspire girls like her, girls who have suffered too much. The least criticism was equal to a hundred of the best compliments. His mind was cruel and unfair; and his vision, lover of his own defects. He was going to the table while his policemen were burned for insecurities; he grabbed pills while his surgical procedures were erased from the books; he swallowed incessantly while the lives of his followers took a course without the same light. She fell evading her responsibility to humanity, avoiding her destiny, turning her back on a future that looked nostalgic at her.

Diagnosis: myopia

Go get your eyes checked. How can you not see that? You need to wear glasses urgently.

«What will be there?», I wondered before a nebula of opaque and poorly defined colors. It was swimming underwater on land as if your eyes couldn't stand that atmosphere and were in dire need of some snorkels. "Come closer if you wish to see." What a painful phrase for a young man whose distance means blindness. It comes slowly, and like any gradual process, you don't notice its presence clearly. Some glasses solve the problem and stop its progression, but that is where thousands of questions arrive: Who was the creator of these complex devices? What will become of those who do not have access to them, of those who have forgotten their sight, who see a totally different universe and there is no one who shares their optics?

Diagnosis: vice

A man who had achieved more than many imagined, but tied to a vice as a child that, even at his age, he had not managed to overcome.

He killed himself day by day and then looked in the mirror and regretted it. How had he fallen into such degradation? Why had he abandoned his cause? It was sad to see how his mind was thinking of nothing else, a mind whose wit and imagination were unmatched; how her hands fell so low for an orgasm, being so good at arousing them in her partners. His eyes were spent watching something dirty on the Internet with so much beauty that there was in reality. His future, according to him, would be bright, but his present was the antagonism of that word. "Reserved prognosis" the doctor said, the truth is that everything depends on him, everything is in his hands. I want to help him, he can be a key piece in the future of humanity.

Diagnosis: Hypothyroidism

She had been fired from her job because of the changes that this stewardess had presented and she arrived imploring the endocrinologist for help.

I have been fired after so much sacrifice. My beautiful skin is now thick and cold; my smiling face became listless; my tongue can hardly sleep in my mouth, preventing it from resting due to the lack of air, my hair visits the ground never to return and my waist stretches with new properties. Where did my energy go? Why does everything I eat accumulate? My breathing has slowed and my heart follows suit. "Someone caused this, someone wants to hurt me," my mind tells me constantly. My face is disfigured, my body is tired, my judgment varies and my life falls apart.

Diagnosis: hyperthyroidism

A man, whose gaze sparkled, with bulging eyes and thin as himself, he didn't know if he was going too fast or life was too slow. He wanted to rest from that whirlwind, so he decided on surgery, as the medication was not working.

-I have to do something! said that bright-eyed man who couldn't sit down. He watched everything in such a way that his eyes wanted to pop out of their sockets. He was sweating without further ado, he could not bear the heat of the environment, his body was an intense summer. His body was going a hundred kilometers per hour, nervous, trembling and afraid of crashing; I couldn't waste time enjoying life. He had spontaneous tachycardia, periodic famines, plenty of food and no body, plenty of food and no profit. Her hair was leaving, as was her patience; the stress threshold had lost all its value; sleep had become the greatest of luxuries and sex no longer appealed to her. The neck betrayed the thyroid, which wanted to export hormones, which wanted to exceed its limits.

Diagnosis: vitiligo

A woman walked with a magnificent character and a Greek attitude, one of those who sit at the top of the Colosseum. No one understood how someone like that could look like that.

Black and white, the zebra of the human kingdom, the breaking of minds small where racism prevails.

—Why homogeneous if there is variety? the body told its army to remove skin cells.

—Let's be the art that represents the diversity of DNA. Do not Cry! -the body said to its owner. -Be the new face of the covers and collapse the superficiality a bit! Show other beings like you that they shouldn't be ashamed of anything! While others are dirt, you include snow; while others are night, in you the day develops; while others only have yin, yang is included in you. You are a beautiful dermatological duality.

Diagnosis: monilia

A relationship had been in trouble. That couple of years and out of a conservative mindset she decided to go to the doctor.

-"My husband wants to kill me." He says that I have betrayed him, that I have infected him with fungus from a sin. Me, who would never do something like that to him, who washes constantly, who is very careful with my hygiene. Why do I have this incessant itching? Why do I expel secretions? What has happened to my private parts that I feel so swollen? Have they done something bad to me, some curse? Has my husband created this farce to get rid of the guilt?

-No ma'am. The fault is of his excess of hygiene, of his extreme care. The perfect physiology of her vagina has been destroyed with so much humidity. You have eliminated the acidity that characterizes it, which kept microorganisms at bay. The monilia has entered his nation without going through customs, and the washes of his aesthetics and pride gave him shelter. And he will continue like this until he understands that washing is once a day, that his physiology is perfect up to a limit.

Diagnosis: cholera

An epidemic was beginning: many had eaten sea fish of dubious origin and were dehydrated in our rooms.

A rascal surfed the waters of the intestine, the white ocean of Hades. How many times can the human go to the bathroom in twenty-four hours? This was the question he always asks himself, the record he longs to break. Dehydration comes in hours; and decomposition, in moments. The fall of one translates into thousands, and the epidemic begins to paint a picture of dirt with the watch on the wrist. What a horrendous image of the choleric! End our ego by showing how fragile we are and how much we need water. The bathroom will be your new home; and toilet paper, your tool of life. It will be a sabotage in the dam of your intestines contaminating everything in its path, with nothing to stop its progress through the rice fields.

Diagnosis: homosexual

A desperate religious man entered the guardhouse asking for help for his son who, according to him, had a fatal disease.

-"How do I cure him, doctor?" It is not normal for a man to be with another man. How do I get rid of this disease?

—Your son is homosexual, and that is not a disease, it is just one more taste.

-No! You and I are not. God forbid. Never will create a family.

-"Your son can adopt, and I'm sure he'll be a great father with his partner

-"What sacrilege is that?" He must have done something to her. He introduced some virus that damaged his brain.

- "I assure you that does not exist."

- "You doctors are fakes. They go around in their smocks and forget about the main problem: the fagots! Those who end the species. Forget diabetes and vaccinations, and get to work on a cure for this disease. Can't you see that I am a suffering father, who will never have a true grandson, a daughter-in-law to take care of my children? Am I doomed to this suffering for life? Help me doctor, I'll pay you anything.

Diagnosis: schizophrenia

He did not understand her, that woman would turn her face away from any bitter-tasting fact that upset her, that was not part of the wonderful world of her imagination.

He looked in the mirror at reality and this was the most unpleasant image he had ever seen in his life: wrinkles from injustice, deformities from laziness, bruises from extreme violence, a body mistreated by hunger, without teeth due to malnutrition, without a prosthesis due to lack of of resources. The image began to speak and she could not believe what she was hearing. How could things like this happen in the world? He closed his eyes and imagined a different being, with golden curls as if wealth abounded; with blue eyes as if the sky did not turn black; with a face that reflected innocence, the one that humanity had lost; with an athletic body that was unaware of the scarcity of food. She was the inconsistency between two parallel worlds, living like Alice in Wonderland, the queen of red hearts in front of her while she closed her eyes thinking that nothing would happen, that the monster would not devour her, that she would never enter its jaws.

Diagnosis: unprotected sex

A woman went to the gynecologist for certain complaints and was diagnosed with an STD. Everything seems to indicate that the husband transmitted it to her.

-"Why does the man betray?"

-"Usually for the sex. A genetic drive towards a stunning woman, someone with large mammary glands; a face socialized by the media to make you believe it's cute; legs made up of muscles, tendons, bones and fat; giant buttocks, an area that is associated with fecal material. They struggle to penetrate a crevice with a particular microbiota, full of secretions, and they want to achieve it even more in a region of excrement. That's in theory, but sex is so primitive and instinctive that it makes you forget about it. Of course, this is in the case of the man, but the same is true of the woman; both are human beings. Sex is something magical with the right person, it is being in a coma from an overdose of endorphins, it is the ideal exercise, it purifies the body of stress and problems, but there are those who sacrifice their emotional stability, their peace, their family and their health for a mischief as dangerous as unprotected sex because, according to them, they feel more. In short, the man convinces the woman to have unprotected sex, ejaculates, puts on his clothes and leaves. One more line for the tiger, one more point for the list of diseases. "What an idiot the human being is."

Diagnosis: attention deficit

A woman, too distracted for her liking, went for help from professionals. The maximum time she had managed to stay focused was three minutes and thirty-four seconds.

—Hello, my name is Alexa and I would like your help, because I can't... Wow, are those all your diplomas? It must be someone very intelligent, doctor... What was he saying? Oh yes, I need your help, because I can't concentrate. Many times I want to achieve some task... What a wonderful landscape in that painting! I have always wanted to go to Paris! As I was saying, I can't focus on any task and it's very frustrating, doctor. My mind leads me through all the streets and I am always late for my destination, if I arrive at all... What is this piece for, doctor? Could you close the window? This way I avoid losing concentration... I want to dedicate hours to what I love. I know that it is the only way to be successful, to achieve something great... What is your barber? I have to admit that I like your haircut, I will suggest it to my brother... I want to be a magnifying glass and not an eye, see the bottom of things and not pass by, feel a good kiss and not go from flower to flower .

The doctor started talking while I was looking at his cactus.

-"So you think you'll make it?"

- "Of course, doctor." "Shit, what did he tell me?"

Diagnosis: cardiac tamponade

The prodigy told that student in shock over the death of their parents, on their knees before their eternal enemy, lost in a place that you could call home.

It was a heart that beat without fear. His muscles were an example of inspiration and his blood filled the entire body of his classroom with encouragement. Healthy, truly healthy, without arrhythmias of errors, without doubt atherosclerosis, with an adequate blood pressure of pride, systole to know its place, diastole to be humble. Her blood got out of control, she escaped from her place and she ended up drowning him herself. He was left weak; everything was so sudden that there was no possible adaptation, it could no longer expand. The psychological arrest had been established upon hearing the news. What else did it all matter? His blood had betrayed him by going to a place where he shouldn't be; life was worth little now. He was saved by a pericardiocentesis performed by trained personnel, his family, his friends, his teachers and all the people he had earned. The blood drained, he was able to breathe, and he came to. Now he had one more reason to meet his goals. He was another, hypertrophied by reality, his coronary network of contacts had increased, his determination had become an unstoppable bomb that did not rest, his flow of ideas convinced millions. He was in a constant fight against the eternal enemy of life, with an eternal devotion for humanity.

Diagnosis: colostomy

A teenager was assaulted and stabbed. They had to rush him to the living room. To save him, they removed a part of his intestines, and when he woke up and became conscious, the doctor explained that he would have to "defecate through his abdomen."

-"Call him what he's a doctor, I'll have to shit in a bag."

"We took a part of you to save you", "you will defecate through the abdomen"... What words to come out of a dream, what consolation when returning from death. He looked in the mirror and swore to take revenge on that cursed reality starting at that very moment. "Call it what it is, doctor, I'll have to shit in a bag." Realistic to the point of being unable to, he would live like that, with certain limitations, with inevitable sorrows. He would eat like this, surrounded at a table, where not everyone would look at him with pleasure, not everyone would resist seeing that. He would make love like this, with a bag of his feces on top of the woman he wanted. He entered inside her like a Spartan and riddled each of her traumas, tortured her insecurities, crucified her regrets, murdered her weakness and returned dragging her strength by the hair. He studied without rest, two hours in the gym and one hour of reading, he went out to parties with his friends and women. Obsessed with being better, with never giving up, every night the same nightmare - "he will have to defecate through his abdomen" -

and what he would reply when getting up: "Call him what he is a doctor, I will have to shit in a bag!".

Diagnosis: burned

An interview was conducted with a firefighter who sacrificed himself for a child and had been left in a delicate situation. His words sounded glorious, but his eyes told a different story.

My skin said goodbye, my muscles abandoned me, my bones remind me of sulfur. A smooth tissue turned into stretch marks, an enviable anatomy regressed into hypotrophy. He was not the same, he had been defeated by the enemy he swore to eliminate. Living example of the word burn that spread through his red body. With areas of pain and others ignorant of it, births of blisters and charred skin, the great walls of Babylon had fallen exposing the city to invaders.

"What will be of my life? I have given it for a child, I have given my job, my happiness, my comfort, my body... All for a child I don't know, who I don't know if he will be a good man. Being honest, I don't know what would have happened if they warned me about what was going to happen, if they had told me the price I would have to pay", said that man with his disfigured face looking in the mirror, following his course leaning on sticks .

Diagnosis: bipolar

A girl visited the psychiatrist. According to her, she couldn't take it anymore between that internal struggle that was disputed daily in her mind between their two personalities. The doctor looked at her and wrote.

The Viking goddess and a cheap prostitute were housed in the same body. One knew her worth and the offerings of those who wanted to possess her, sitting on her throne of self-esteem, shaped by determination and will. It was the first in the fights. Holding an ax can also be done by a woman. Last to sleep, she had to protect the home. He did not depend on anything or anyone, hunting, fishing, searching and building. The ego knelt down and knowledge praised her. She was a Viking in all her being, rough in character and gentle in manner, with an ax and flowers, with a cold look and a joyous smile, with blood on her cheeks and kisses on her mouth. The other lived crying under every situation. Melancholy was her best friend; the complaints, his writing. Drug addict of a little affection, dependent on a few words. Disgust gives and disgust receives, stressed and withered acclaiming something that only she possesses. She vomited her pride and he didn't even look at her, she defecated her shame in the pipes of a forgotten city. He asks for a penny for an hour with his body, he asks for a penny so that they take pity on his situation. Dressed in insecurities, with dishonorable heels, she goes to the brothel of her destiny, where she is brutally raped by reality, while the chains of her thoughts keep her tied to the bed.

Diagnosis: Acquired immunodeficiency virus

He was a patient who was diagnosed with AIDS, his condition already showed signs of the disease and he didn't know much about it, so he asked the doctor.

He was a highly skilled politician, raised and trained by the worst of disease society, by the pathological underworld. He came to power and the first thing he paid attention to was the T CD4 Special Forces squad, in charge of the internal affairs of the Corporal Government. His word spread by thousands, his ideology multiplied. Little by little, he lowered the squad's priorities: fewer hours of training, ignoring calls that were not important, more months of vacation... The effective squad became a group of donut-eating officers, while the streets were dominated and destroyed by the family. "opportunist". Candidiasis managed the bets on the mouth and vagina; Tuberculosis, slavery in the lung; Kaposi's sarcoma drug dealing all over the skin. All of them responded to a single master and lord to whom they owed their success. The virus, after seeing how it ended that government, got out of the chair and got on its jet towards the secretions, towards a new government.

Diagnosis: reading epilepsy

An avid reader, worried about bringing on epilepsy, though it only arose from reading: his most exquisite habit. He visited the neurologist, who exposed his disease.

Two books a month. It was a pleasure to turn the page, to have more and more knowledge. A book arrived that changed his life: 1984. Ignorance is strength. The brain used as a weapon what was more of a warning. Like any dictatorship, it would eliminate any risk to her, anyone who knew too much. He issued an order—"No reading!"—and since all orders go unpunished, he deployed the neural army. The eyes, seeing something dangerous, suffered neural discharges that made the whole body pay for it. The organs began to hate him and he had no choice but to close in on himself and live in the darkness of ignorance, fearing knowledge. That man, requested by his wisdom, began to decline. I got less and less qualified jobs, less stable. I was falling from the digital age into obscurantism, believing what the masses said. He was docile, with almost no vocabulary. There was a phrase that he repeated every night: "Ignorance is power."

Diagnosis: alcoholism

A fully rehabilitated man next to his daughter. From far It looked like she had helped a lot.

-It feels? he asked.

—Finishing off the mafia, the best thing in the world. You feel invincible.

-Mafia?

The great families of organized crime, Tequila, Ron and Don Vino, dominated the Government under the shadow of problems and concerns. «Another drink, from habit to vice». They were thieves of great fortunes, respect, dreams, life. Boss of bosses was Alcohol, destroyer of bodies and minds. He had politicians in his pocket like the brain blackmailed with delusions. Cirrhosis frightened the liver that it could hardly degrade, it gave promises of recovery to broken hearts. It was the only outlet offered to the marginalized. He dominated everything, master and lord of every cell in the body. He bribed justice, the family ignored him, society withdrew, doctors ignored him. Few, very few came out of them. Those with wealth to pay the debt were free, people who did not give up, who possessed unconditional support and a will of steel. There are still free beings who escape from the worst of families, from the liquid claw, from the ethyl government.

Diagnosis: vesicouterine fistula

That woman barely made it to the hospital. After delivery, shame devoured her and, even so, her family brought her in for surgery, to fix his situation once and for all, the one that stole his life.

It was the worst union of all, a wonder followed by a tragedy. She made too much effort in that delivery. Two different paths came together, and shame, together with disgust, joined hands. She has urine on her private parts, an unpleasant smell, impregnated like the best of perfumes. Hidden in her room, she doesn't even want to talk about it. She is estranged from her partner; She doesn't think she can satisfy him, she doesn't think he understands her. The isolation, the secrets and the justifications for those who do not see it stand out. Scratching from irritation, scratch infections; the vicious cycle of decay. The vagina is already disgusted, the bladder is empty, the person does not know what to do. How to go to the hospital in those conditions? How to ask for help with an unmentionable problem? How can that proud organ recover? Withered, degraded and tasteless, she rises half dead and comes to see us. She doesn't think anything worse will happen, she doesn't think we can help her.

Diagnosis: diabetes insipidus

On the way I observed a person who was drinking water as if This was the most precious asset on the planet, and he went to the bathroom as if it were incontinence. The endocrinologist took care of his case with a simple substance.

-"Drink, I'm dehydrated." —This was the advice of the body to that patient.

The hypothalamus, angry with the kidney, stopped producing vasopressin and the whole body paid for that conflict. There is no saving, only spending; it is the wasteful mentality of the kidney that spends all the water that reaches its pockets, forcing its owner to go into debt to satisfy his tastes. The owner became a slave, and the water, the currency of life. "Baby, I'm dehydrated. Pee and drink, you don't want to go into shock, feel cold or pass out, so drink." Nights are not for resting, they are for going to the bathroom. Always have a little water on hand; no matter the source, it's drink or die. He is a miniature dry planet, a constant stream of liquid, someone aware of the importance of water.

-"Give me that hormone!" he yelled desperately. Save me at once!

Diagnosis: tuberculosis

A not very young girl was looking for her medicines. The truth it is that they were many, since the treatment was of six months. I trembled at hear the expression that said to the doctor:

-"You don't know how much I want to finish the treatment. Has passed Long time since I don't kiss my daughter.

It produces red and encapsulated sputum, its size is inversely proportional to its resistance, it has imperialist spirits, it does not want to be local, it wants to be systemic. A close friend of AIDS, they usually share patients, they usually go hand in hand. She is slow and crushing, a cunning commander. By the time she is discovered, she has already taken over the kingdom. It gives us sweat baths at night, coughing at every moment, always feeling down. Thinness is established prevailing, fever is not usually important. Its appetite is voracious and the lung is not enough to contain it. It inflames anything: pericardium, meninges and bones. The air is usually their medium and contagion is always abundant. Saliva is your tram; the kisses, their private jets. You must take strong pills in large doses for a long time. A raffle was held at the Istanbul Pyramid. The exaggeration of your cure, you heal the lung, but you damage other organs. He is a lover of the worst places: jail, overcrowding and alcoholics, the worst of humanity.

What a bacillus. The day will come when everyone will fear him when he becomes incurable.

Diagnosis: bulimia

A teenager, who barely ate, her mother brought her to the psychiatrist, but it seemed more like a case from the nutritionist. obsessed With being a model, she had to keep her body to the limit, she had to take it to the extreme.

Mother, can't you see that I'm fat? In this society, if you are not thin, you are not valued, and men do not look at you. Mother, I have come a long way, my ribs and bones are showing, I can already see my joints. Mother, have you changed the mirrors? I look wide in all of them. Is my sacrifice to lose weight not enough? I guess I have to try harder. Mother, I have failed you, I have eaten everything in the kitchen, I could not stand such hunger. Mother, I am sorry for my actions and I will do anything to make amends: I will vomit, I will exercise or I will take laxatives. Mother, I am dizzy, my legs are shaking, my hair is falling out, my cavities are increasing and my skin is dry. Mother, it's already more than two days a week for more than three months. Don't you think you should do something about it? Mother… I need help!

Diagnosis: sterile

That gynecologist did not know what to do to have children. She had already tried all the methods: from in vitro fertilization to not very scientific procedures. It was presented in our office on the day of the Mothers

What can I do, doctor, if I want to be a mother, if I want to bring life into my womb, if I want to feel its little kicks? What do I do doctor if I have disappointed my husband as a couple, my family as a daughter and humanity as a species? Do I only count on my beauty? Am I only good for sex? How can I create a home if I can't even bring a child to life? I have everything, doctor: money, comfort, love, and they deny me this out of hand. I, who have always protected myself, who have always been a correct woman. Envy corrodes my soul when I see a mother and her child. It pains me to be ignorant of that feeling. How ironic, doctor. A specialist when it comes to bringing life into the world, so that I cannot create it. Yuck altruism! I would give the life of ten to have one, lose my title, be fired, as long as I have a child, as long as they congratulate me on Mother's Day.

Diagnosis: deafness

A music-loving woman had suffered from an illness who stole his ear, his job and his life.

What do you say, that the void has taken over my life, that the cochlear balance has been broken forever? The music didn't even say goodbye, it didn't even give my tympanic membrane a fucking kiss. I miss the sound so much in this galaxy of silence… From the notes of my violin to the cry of a baby. Why take away my favorite meaning, stealing my career, challenging me like Beethoven, leaving me without my nightly peace of magnificent sound, without the inspiration of musical notes? It's almost inhuman that I'm forgetting my mother's sweet voice scolding me, my daughter's rebelliousness in her words, the support that came from my husband's mouth... It's not the same without his deep and high pitched tones. I am learning sign language so that I can listen with my eyes, so that when I see each gesture, I don't shed my tears.

Diagnosis: High blood pressure

In the dining room, a man was taking out pills next to lunch; He had to control his hypertension. Although looking closely, it did not seem Seriously: his plate and his appearance were not healthy at all.

- "Too fast for my liking." I don't know how much I can hold on, -said the blood vessels.

The heart and the kidney looked at each other; one afraid of not being enough; the other, to vomit albumin. The brain did wonders to prevent stroke. Hypertension is here to stay, smoking with style. His belly protruded from his shirt dirty with salt and grease; genetics supported his decisions. The eyes did not want to look at her, they were a little red, and the nose, feeling her stench, began to bleed. Thinking of her brought pain.   -"Refrain from your emotions. I have broken the valve and the measure. You will be a slave to pills and doctors, checking what will always be high. I don't kill, I am the snake that expels you from paradise for biting the apple, for disobeying orders. I am too much for you, for your body and for your organs, the most terrible physical law implanted in your life, the ironic wear and tear of speed. Too much pressure for such a small vessel, where it's only a matter of time... before you explode.

Diagnosis: locked-in syndrome

An older gentleman wanted to dive. He saved up and went to fulfill his dream. For the moment, he lost all capacity: his body did not respond not at all, his mind was still intact.

I wanted to dive and they got me a suit made of my own skin, just right for me. I went to the Pacific, far from all humanity, and in those deep waters I jumped into solitude. As I fell, I saw some magnificently colored fish. They came from everywhere, brightening my day. Over time they were fewer, larger and even became violent. He could see her teeth of anger and contempt. Deep down they could be defined as sea monsters, they had deformed, they were gigantic. They could devour me in one bite and, although some tried, they ended up spitting on me because of the bad taste of prison, of rust, of years in prison. Everything became so dark that I could hardly see and my thought did not change: "What a strange metamorphosis that of those fish, what more abrupt changes the human being can experience."

Diagnosis: atrial fibrillation

A man fell to the ground in the middle of the guardhouse, and the doctors came to his rescue. After learning the cause, a defibrillator brought him back to life.

The atria went on strike and the myocytes were tired of working so many hours straight for so little adenosine triphosphate. They took up arms against the sinoatrial node and began to contract when they wanted, subjugated under the supposed perfect order of the body that was currently a dishonor, exposed to pathological conditions. All in the same boat, all on the same strike, each one rowing in their own way and, therefore, they were not going anywhere. The contractions did not take place, the infusion stopped, the body paid the price. Such a strike would wipe out the entire country; The authorities had to do something. They were given a corrective shock to remind everyone of their place, to remind everyone of their role. You were born myocardium, don't expect to die neuron. They could not face the technological superiority of the human being, so they lowered their heads waiting for the body to weaken again, waiting for the propitious moment for the next strike.

Diagnosis: Compartment syndrome

An accident had occurred: a patient's leg had I've been under a lot of rubble for a long time.

They locked up too many cells in a prison and the tension could be breathed in the environment. The first days morale prevailed and they divided the few resources equally. Then the robberies, fights and murders began. Too little food for too many heads. Survival was the law; kindness, a weakness. Cellular debris sins reigned. Cannibalism began, they created groups to protect themselves, they returned to savagery with each passing day. They were released, and when society opened its doors to them, it did not recognize them; they no longer saw the rest of the world as their equals. Before they were his brothers and now they were his food, and taking their spears they went to the attack. An irreversible combat broke out, an invasion of toxins towards a perfect homeostasis.

Diagnosis: renal colic

The pain was unbearable, to the point of fainting. She didn't know where to put her dignity or her screams, the pills barely had an effect, and all because of a stone in the wrong place.

-"Don't you listen?" I want to go out! said that calcic sum embedded in a path too narrow for her. He pounded incessantly, extending his dominance. Nerves scribbled the information—pain, pain, pain—and some even fainted from exhaustion. It was synonymous with a birth, since it had to expel a being, it had unbearable pain, and after leaving, everyone was happy. The positions made fun of the patient; no one was willing to help him. The water was an abandoned woman that now the man desperately claimed. -Kick it! said that hopeless soul.

-Get it out of my body! —And there goes the stone, making its way into a new territory, advancing at the expense of the pain of others, causing tears without noticing them, with the sole purpose of leaving, with the desire to fulfill its goal.

Diagnosis: chronic renal failure

A man, who needed an urgent kidney transplant, was undergoing hemodialysis. We started talking and I he said his urea had said "here I stay!" without caring about the opinion of the kidney.

The kidney was tired and the urea took over after being an expat life. Now he could stay, and he vowed to take revenge and help anyone who was expelled by the kidneys. The fluids were accumulating. He made great cardiac pathological alliances, and hypertension and insufficiency knelt on his throne. Potassium was finally free to roam the blood. I spent hours planning arrhythmias. The anemia came home with its characteristic fatigue, and the erythropoietic guard had already been eliminated. They broke huge dams, and the edema could swim sharply in the lungs. Phosphate finally beat calcium in a pulse, and the parathyroids got their gym, renal osteoporosis, vascular calcifications. Metabolic acidosis came with its pathognomonic respiration, with its manifest pH. It achieved damage to large uremic targets, encephalopathies and pericarditis. It was the revenge of those exiled by a dictatorship of organic perfection.

Diagnosis: acute myocardial infarction

It was a couple of doctors, now older. The woman had suffered He had a heart attack and was recovering, and by his side was his partner. She called him "atheromatous plaque", and the truth is that she did not understand why.

An innocent woman's heart had been broken, and she vowed never to feel anything for the male species again. Her beauty was too conspicuous, but she created a warrior with an indestructible heart, a heart that wasn't willing to die for anyone. Someone willing to do anything arrived, with a different strategy: LDL —low-density lipoproteins or bad cholesterol— was his key. With his details he was infiltrating his arteries, with his jokes he forgot his exercises in indifference, and his insistence lowered his metabolism. After a year of trying, an atheromatous plaque formed; finally he accepted the appointment and presented symptoms of angina: a chest pressure that he did not know if it was due to fear or adrenaline. The palpitations were symptoms that something would change. The lack of air awoke because of an atmosphere that he had forgotten. After such an incident, she became concerned, resumed her healthy lifestyle—for her—and eliminated it from her diet, no matter how much she liked it. Time passed and, as fate would have it, he suffered an accident; As fate would have it, he was in the ER. He took care of her daily, pampered her like no one else, treated her like royalty. When she was discharged, she appeared with a bouquet of flowers saying everything she felt and, at once, that atheromatous plaque ruptured, unleashing a cascade of emotions. All of the above, but stronger. His nightmare, his forgotten dream, came true. There was no time for cardiopulmonary resuscitation for that toxic friend, there was no stent for that artery that irrigated his unhappiness, there were no drugs that would reverse such a situation. That woman who didn't believe in anything died, who wouldn't give any chance, who would never fall in love again.

Diagnosis: multiple sclerosis

A patient, who had lost many of her body functions, visited the neurologist, who told her that her brain was gradually losing control of her body.

The government did not pay its army well and it was already dissatisfied, planning a coup. He decided to cut communications, imprisoned the mayors, state secretaries and main leaders, and they could no longer give orders. He couldn't speak well, his best spokesmen were under arrest. The Sports Council was exploited in arduous tasks to weaken them, and the muscles, not knowing what to do, produced uncoordinated and meaningless movements, contracted or rigid from fear. The brain could not reason, it was in the middle of the civil war. The Brain Internal Service snipers were taken out, and the corporal nation lost much of their vision. Government poets and writers had their books burned; to the painters, their works. There could be nothing to make you feel anything; neither pain nor heat nor touch. The army planned to end the government's morale, incontinence, impotence and loss of libido. There was nothing to do. The defense became the weapon, the problem had no escape. The division was a law; and unity, a utopia.

Diagnosis: retinitis pigmentosa

The ophthalmologist examined a woman, who only saw towards the center as if she were looking through a tunnel, and her entire retina was colonized by spots.

He was a lover of the most beautiful landscapes and could not stand anything that ruined the view. He lived complaining about everything that got in the way of his field of vision. The DNA, tired of his regrets, planned to carry out his wishes. They searched for a brush and became painters of those who dull colors, of those who censor ideas, as effective as they are indelible. To each image that did not like, braz!, a brushstroke. That symphony of complaints was a concert of the dark. The micro ended up becoming macro. The vision began to decline, Guanina was smiling and the person was worried. How odd! What he asked for was being fulfilled. The woman sought help, although there was not much to do: Cytosine had already acquired the brush; Adenina, the painting; and Timina had paid for the course and they would not stop until they finished their work, until the canvas was totally dark.

Diagnosis: eschar

An old nurse was in the room where she worked so much, and came back in the same state in which he treated his patients as karmic thing.

-Fuck! Can't you see that it hurts? said that old woman as they lifted her out of bed.

«My skin has exposed me to everyone as how unpleasant the human body is, my fat shows off and my muscles are not even hidden, the sheets stick to my body and the pain causes screams. So many that I cured and now I understand what they felt", she said to herself, while they performed a cure on her, while they entered her withered body without the slightest compassion or kindness.

How far have I fallen? How unpleasant I feel. The mirror is torture; the cures, a hell; I have morale on the floor. The irony of life returns to its zero point. Before I was the insensitive one who cleaned a stranger, now a stranger cleans me insensitively.

Diagnosis: gangrene

A diabetic had pricked his foot with a nail and was never treated. After a while, he came to the room desperate for his member, that it had changed color.

My skin is changing and I don't know what to do. A cold fire is dyeing it black; It doesn't hurt, it just kills all life in its path. Firefighters in red try to stop the expansion with jets of blood, logistics do everything possible to provide resources to the victims and the Police are activated to catch any arsonist. The army of death advances through my member playing its depraved flute and the flies respond to the call; their larvae will fulfill the objective. The smell of a battlefield is felt on my leg, the putrefaction is palpable and death is seen while being alive. My breakdown, still conscious, still with my heart beating. Amputation is imminent; He had that word tattooed on his leg. Nobody would think that a simple nail would trigger this, nobody thinks that the worst will happen to him, that he will be part of a negative statistic.

Diagnosis: prostate cancer

A seventy-year-old man came in concerned about his symptoms, because these were reminiscent of a disease. We explained to him what had to be done a rectal examination, and he refused. He said that since he was fifty he had to do it, but that it would never happen... even after thinking about it.

The rebels rose up and their followers multiplied by the day; more and more areas were conquered. The micturition dripping was a sign of supply cuts by them. They caused urinary retention, difficulty in eliminating waste; they wanted the dead to create epidemics on the battlefield. They attacked at night and their symptoms shone; the nocturia showed up at those hours. Notices of annual reviews, but this one refused. The corrupted smile of the general of the rebels could be seen; they had given him permission to continue his conquest. The years passed and the manhood of an irresponsible man was worth more than his health. He ignored the war that was going through his body and the ambition of the rebels was not limited to the prostate. New allies arrived: anemia, weight loss, exhaustion, and red-hot blood in your urine. At this stage, the worry was bigger than his masculine pride, and his refusal had alarmed all his loved ones, his inability to overcome a prejudice had killed his body.

Diagnosis: cataracts

A woman visited the ophthalmologist, because she could barely see. I was older and yet he retained a mysterious charm. I loved gray according to his clothing and it seems that his eyes wanted to join the group.

The optical city was like Atlantis, a magnificent development, the paradise of the entire planet, the illumination of biological technology. The gods, infatuated with their power, did not want them to continue enjoying such views, and their eyes had enjoyed it too much, it was time to change things. They sent a storm, and the clear sky turned gray, the transparent waters turned opaque, and a waterfall seemed to gush out of the clouds, flooding everything in its path, suffocating everything beautiful. The city became an underwater ruin and families were divided, never to see each other. They couldn't find food or salvation. What was once light is now shadow; what you once cherished, you hardly remember now. The image of such a scenario was seen from a submarine by those who managed to escape. They saw it as an opaque and distorted image through glass that was too fogged up, through glass that needed to be replaced.

Diagnosis: intraparenchymal hemorrhage

A man brought to the ER was found slumped in the floor eating a hamburger and Coca-Cola. Your blood pressure It was high and together with other exams we arrived at...

Hypertension and his team planned a terrorist act - let it rain blood on the brain nation. Hidden in the sewers, they planted bombs in the main pipes. They thought to overwhelm the city. At zero hour they all detonated together.

Boom! The head pounded and the headache was unrelenting. The city fell into chaos and lost its balance. It rained blood, and a red cloud appeared in the meteorological centers of the cerebral cortex. The population reacted differently, some numb and paralyzed, some could not see due to the impact and others could not swallow due to the trauma. Some people didn't speak for days. No one understood why such an atrocity had happened. The act fulfilled its objective, according to what Hypertension said: to implant fear. They were no longer the same: listless, lethargic or in a coma. They informed the Government and it announced that the cause was not known, that it could not do anything. His hands were tied; he himself had introduced it to the city and could not say such a thing in the media.

Diagnosis: disappointment dyscrasia

In my walk I found a man lying down, without any company, as if waiting for death. Seeing that image, I took pity him and went to talk. He told me about his life and the reason for his loneliness, and he asked me as a favor to write about it, about parents who ignore their children.

He was alone in bed, waiting for a transfusion. Sometimes they visited him, but his blood group was not in any of them, and although they tried to help him, the doctors said that it was not the same, that the genetic component was missing. Blood dyscrasia was his disease, dyscrasia of disappointments. Her own immune system had ravaged her red blood cells with helplessness and little attention. His blood, his own blood, that which is transmitted from generation to generation, had been destroyed, and his remains were metabolized with indifference and expelled into oblivion in the worst possible way. Over time, the bone marrow couldn't do any more and stopped producing. There were no longer even small, immature globules with the causeless intention of saving what was left. Deterioration took hold of him, organ failure, degeneration and more. Sadness gnawed at him when he saw other patients how they could do it and he couldn't. suffered. His blood left his body and he no longer had the strength to take it back. I finished writing the story, turned and left, knowing that I would never see that man

alone in bed again, waiting for a transfusion.

Diagnosis: dementia

An older gentleman in the waiting room didn't know how he got there. We were hoping that his relatives had seen the publications made by the hospital about that patient suffering from dementia...

¿Will I remember who I am, my family and my friends? It hurts sometimes not to remember my son's face, not to know if my wife kissed me, to go out and ask myself "did I say goodbye?", to be in the middle of a task and not know where I am going, to ask the same thing thousands of times until they end up screaming and not knowing the reason for their words and their insults. The directions are confusing to me and the faces are the same To some, a light gives them an idea, but it takes it away from me. I don't remember much of my life, I don't remember much of what I do. Have I been a good father? Did I help who I could? What memories will they have of me? My words are not the same and my help is not needed. I can no longer put my grandson's shirt on, nor write how I feel, nor eat with cutlery; I don't know if it's me anymore. The mind became Judas and my body follows the rhyme. I don't want my family to hate me, to be left in the care of a caregiver, admitted to a hospital until ulcers appear on my body, until an infection steals my life.

Diagnosis: ventricular fibrillation

That man survived the heart attack; the truth is that he did nothing to avoid it, it seemed that he wanted to die. Within a few hours, the herald of death took his life.

The cerebral Government took too absurd measures and the economy of the body could no longer hold up. The town was nothing short of rebellion. The infarction occurred, the feeding of the myocytes was suspended for days while the neurons continued to enjoy glucose delicacies; they didn't care. The people took up arms ready for anything. They would rather die than bear such injuries. He forgot about the atria and went to overthrow the ventricular army, the one that maintained order so that the Government would not fall, the one with great muscular power. The nodes gave speeches to stop them, human technology spared no resources to prevent it. "The revolution of anarchy is already imposed and there is not much we can do" was what the news on the EKG channel said. The brain said: "The country will go to ruin! Don't you see what you are doing? They were a bunch of hypocrites. They suffered nothing from the misery of that people who did not stop working, who kept a corrupt government afloat. Blinded by hatred, they imposed a national strike and the allied nations did their best to help, but to no avail. In the end the body fell on fire, cremated, for underestimating his people.

Diagnosis: death

A doctor was kneeling before a bed. his patient was in a coma and supported life only by devices and not by her. Unfortunately, it was his daughter, a recently graduated doctor. Asked to the doctor how I could help you:

-*"It's impossible," he told me.*

For some reason I saw his soul in bed, and I asked him what was death like

-Death? I don't care about that, but I miss life so much. If they gave me one more day, I don't know how many things I would do. There is so much I would like to know! So many answers that I don't know! I would practice my profession like never before, I would listen to my tutor's every word, I would encourage a patient, I would save a life and I would hug my parents, even if my gown is dirty or I am dead tired. That day I would exercise a little, I would dress sexy, I would walk slim and I would smile more. I would donate a part of my money to whoever needs it, I would give gifts to children with cancer, I would feed the street dogs, I would surprise a homeless person with a ticket and I would provide the favorite treats of my loved ones. I would try the forbidden, I would do what I want, from kissing the boy I like to asking for forgiveness from someone who deserves it; I would go to the

127

beach, to the movies, to the museum and to the ballet, since I could never appreciate them. I would get a tattoo that says "Live big, dream bigger and love like never before!" on the left clavicle, near the heart, visible enough to serve as a lesson to all of you. It would be me, without lies, without fear, without caring about the rest of the opinions. It would be me! With the stretch marks of my soul, with my spontaneous madness, with my overcome traumas. He would say "yes or no," with the pride of the gods and without the remorse of the damned. I would make love with someone special, I would treat myself to a few orgasms, some kisses and an interesting conversation under the covers. I would choose people not for cheap superficialities, but for how they make me feel, for what they transmit to me. It doesn't matter if they are staggering lies, wild ideas, or impossible conspiracies. I would read a good book, the kind that you can touch, turn the page, cross out and point to, the kind that you give away after reading to a soul that needs that knowledge. I would write something cute but realistic to every doctor. Exact! To every doctor! So that they don't forget that they should enjoy that coffee that lifts them up, those smiles on duty, the thanks of a dying person who has nothing else to offer, the nonsense of a friend while they study, feeling on the palate hospital food that barely tastes like anything. I would get strength from anywhere to savor the blessings of life, even when my body yells at me to rest. How am I going to rest? Death hates me. I wear white and she wears black, I frustrate her work and she mine; a fight as unequal as it is eternal, a scythe against what is in hand. In the end he will win and I will continue to save lives. In the end he will take revenge and I will continue living. At the end it will ask me:

-¿why you did?

And I will answer:

-I'm in love!